Hypertension

A guide to assessment and management

A history of
hypertension

A guide to the major discoveries in blood, circulation and blood pressure

© 2002 Bladon Medical Publishing Limited
12 New Street, Chipping Norton, Oxfordshire OX7 5LJ
Tel: +44 (0)1608 644436 Fax: +44 (0)1608 646166

E-mail: info@bladonmedical.com
Internet: www.bladonmedical.com

First published 2002

British Library Cataloguing-in-Publication Data. A catalogue record
of this title is available from the British Library.

ISBN 1-904218-01-6

Poulter, N, Kirby, M
Hypertension: A guide to assessment and management

Printed by
Grafiche IGC S.R.L., 25128 Brescia, Zona Industriale,
Via A. Grandi, 29, Italy

Distributed by
Plymbridge Distributors Ltd., Estover Road, Plymouth PL6 7PY, UK

Disclaimer

Hypertension

A guide to assessment and management

Neil Poulter MB BS MSc FRCP
*Professor of Preventive Cardiovascular Medicine,
Cardiovascular Studies Unit, Imperial College School of
Medicine at St Mary's, London, UK*

Michael Kirby MB BS LRCP MRCS FRCP
*Family Practitioner, The Surgery, Letchworth, UK and
Director, HertNet (The Hertfordshire Primary Care
Research Network), Hertfordshire, UK*

A history of hypertension

A guide to the major discoveries in blood, circulation and blood pressure

BLADON
MEDICAL
PUBLISHING

Contents

Contents

A history of hypertension

Hypertension – persistently high arterial blood pressure – is common in developed societies, affecting around one-quarter of the population.

Raised blood pressure shows no specific clinical manifestations until target organ damage develops in the vasculature of the heart, eyes, kidneys and brain. As the single most important risk factor for stroke and one of the main risk factors for coronary heart disease, hypertension is the most common indication for chronic lifelong drug treatment.

The history of the growth in understanding of this 'silent killer' and its role in disease, particularly in the past century, has been one in which different elements of scientific endeavour have contributed to an evolving knowledge base that has moved from mysticism, through observation into the realm of experimental intervention. Anatomists, physiologists, biochemists, physicists, physicians, pharmacists and most recently epidemiologists and molecular biologists have all contributed to our current understanding of hypertension and its treatment.

Hypertension

A guide to assessment and management

Hypertension is one of the most common cardiovascular conditions encountered in primary care, and the consequences of hypertension – strokes, renal disease and coronary heart disease – are major causes of incapacity and death.

Hypertension is, however, an ideal subject for preventive medicine initiated in primary care. Early action to identify and treat hypertension can prevent the longer-term complications of this disease.

This pocket guide summarizes current opinion and guidance about the management of hypertension, including:

- diagnosis
- risk assessment
- treatment options

Historical perspectives

The ancient world

In early times, disease was demonized as the result of supernatural forces, its interpretation largely omen-based and treatment based on mystic spells or empirical remedies. Understanding of the human body and its mechanisms in general, and of cardiovascular anatomy in particular, grew with the development of western civilization but for many centuries remained intimately bound up with, and sometimes impeded by, religious beliefs.

The ancient Egyptians believed that well-being was determined by both earthly and supernatural forces, and that illness was due to evil spirits entering the body and consuming the individual's 'vital substance'. The importance of the heart as the seat of the soul is shown by the fact that embalmers would remove the organs of the body through small incisions but leave the heart in place.

Surviving documents suggest that the ancient Egyptians had a reasonable grasp of cardiovascular anatomy. The Edwin Smith Papyrus (c. 1600 BC) is an inventory of case reports on various injuries and wounds and their prognosis and treatment. It describes the heart as being the centre of a system of vessels that extend peripherally throughout the body.

Clinical assessment

Assessing risk in hypertension

The objective of hypertension treatment is to prevent complications such as stroke, renal failure and coronary heart disease, not merely to lower blood pressure. For this reason, guidelines of hypertension management emphasize the importance of considering a patient's overall cardiovascular risk.

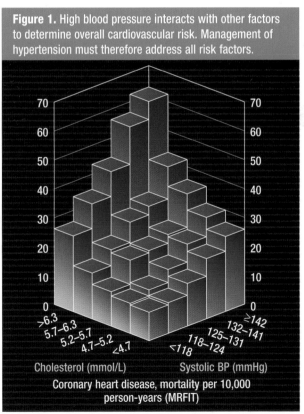

Figure 1. High blood pressure interacts with other factors to determine overall cardiovascular risk. Management of hypertension must therefore address all risk factors.

Cholesterol (mmol/L) Systolic BP (mmHg)

Coronary heart disease, mortality per 10,000 person-years (MRFIT)

Despite making the link between the pulse and the heart, it does not describe the mechanism of the circulation or what it is distributing. The ancient Egyptians believed that air was conveyed to the heart and from there to the other organs of the body. The magical properties of the blood are mentioned in the Ebers Papyrus (c. 1550 BC), which also includes spells and incantations for dealing with various diseases.

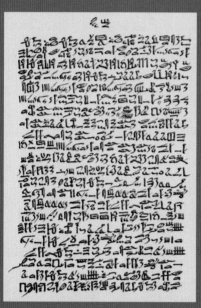

A section of the Ebers payrus refering to the heart and blood vessels

Although Greek culture was heavily influenced by Egyptian ideas and beliefs, medicine became increasingly separated from religion and based more on observation. Nearly 2500 years ago, the Greek physician Hippocrates (460–377 BC) dissected animals and developed a limited

Clinical work-up

Most patients with hypertension have no overt symptoms. A thorough clinical history and physical examination are therefore essential starting points for effective management of the condition.

Lifestyle

Environmental factors such as diet, alcohol, smoking and physical exercise are important influences and should be inquired about during the history-taking.

- A diet high in saturated fats and refined sugars, or with a high proportion of processed food, is associated with increased risk of cardiovascular disease.
- A high alcohol intake is closely related to high blood pressure. This association is independent of age, sex, cigarette smoking or salt consumption.
- Cigarette smoking is an independent risk factor for cardiovascular disease and interacts strongly with other cardiovascular risk factors such as hypertension.
- High salt intake is associated with hypertension. Patients should be asked if they consume large quantities of salt by adding it to food or by eating large amounts of processed foods, which have a high salt content.
- Regular moderate physical exercise can help to reduce cardiovascular risk. Patients should be asked about their exercise patterns.

understanding of cardiac anatomy – he identified four chambers within the heart and showed that the aortic and pulmonary valves opened in only one way. However, he stated that health depended on the balance of the four humours – blood, phlegm, yellow bile and black bile – an idea that was to persist for more than 2000 years.

This theory held that bile and phlegm were harmful as they were exuded in sickness. Blood was considered to be the fount of life and, observing that it was expelled from the body during nosebleeds and menstruation, Hippocratic teaching devised the practice of bloodletting (phlebotomy), which persisted for several centuries.

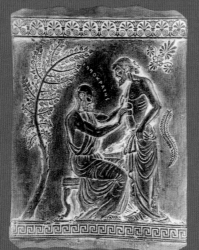

The Greek physician Hippocrates treating a patient

Although Hippocratic medicine perceived disease as a disturbance of the affected individual's health, it made little attempt to

Additional risk

Enquire about the following conditions which affect the blood pressure and/or cardiovascular risk:

- Age
- Smoking habits
- Alcohol consumption
- Physical activity
- Concomitant medication
- Past and current history of coronary heart disease or cerebrovascular disease
- Diabetes
- Lipid disorders
- Oral contraceptive use
- Respiratory illness (especially asthma or chronic obstructive airways disease)
- Recreational drug usage
- Family history

Patient history

The patient's history may give clues to the presence of secondary causes of hypertension. Enquire about:

- past renal disease
- vascular complications of hypertension.

Women patients should be questioned about:

- history of pre-eclampsia or pregnancy-related hypertension.

understand the functioning of the body. Later Greeks such as Aristotle (384–322 BC) became more systematic in their observation of nature, usually of animals, attempting to explain everything in relation to its purpose. He noted that the heart had three chambers connected to the lungs, and made no distinction between arteries and veins. Despite noting that the heart was fundamental to life, Aristotle thought that blood was a nutrient absorbed by the blood vessels from the intestines.

During the Alexandrian era, dissection of condemned criminals was permitted, which fostered an understanding of anatomy and physiology.

Erasistratus (330–255 BC) investigated the valves of the heart and proposed a system by which arteries and veins were connected, thus anticipating the discovery of the capillary system. Praxagorus (340 BC) distinguished arteries from veins, but he believed (like Erasistratus) that air (or pneuma) was conveyed from the lungs to the left side of the heart in arteries (the word is derived from the Greek for air) and from the heart to the other organs of the body through the aorta and other arteries. While the arteries arose from the heart, veins were thought to arise from the liver to carry blood created from digested food to the rest of the body. His student Herophilus (335–280 BC) noted the different structures of arteries and veins, and showed that the arteries contained blood and not air.

Family history It should be fairly easy to identify a family history of hypertension if the patient can recall instances of premature death, heart attack, or stroke in their relatives. More extensive questioning may be needed, however, if the patient does not recall such events clearly.

A family history of hyperlipidaemia or diabetes is relevant as these interact with hypertension to increase overall risk of cardiovascular diseases. A family history of diabetes is important for the same reason.

Adult polycystic renal disease – a recognised cause of secondary hypertension – is inherited as a Mendelian dominant condition.

Figure 2. A typical family tree with hypertension in the father (who died of a stroke), showing the variable occurrence of a raised blood pressure in the children.

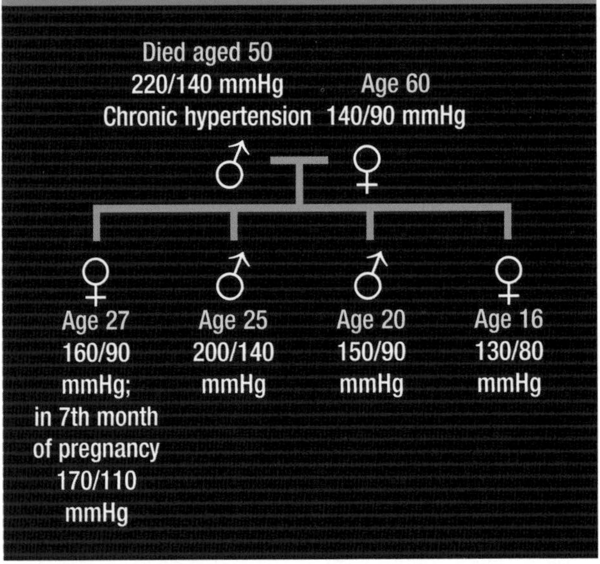

Greek notions of medicine permeated the Mediterranean region throughout the Roman era. Claudius Galen (129–199), a physician from Pergamon, fused practical, clinical observations with the theoretical legacy of Hippocrates, reflecting the somewhat mystical notions of his predecessors.

Galen was a medical scientist who dissected apes, pigs, sheep and goats, as dissection of humans was no longer permitted. He believed that blood was made in the liver incorporating ingested foods, and was transported through veins both to the body carrying natural spirits that supported growth and nutrition and to the right side of the heart. Blood passed from the right to the left side of the heart through invisible pores in the interventricular septum, where it was mixed with air from the lungs.

Renaissance... the break with Galen

As a highly influential physician, Galen's views persisted long after his death. Indeed, right through to the Middle Ages, medical knowledge relied on his teachings and those of Hippocrates, hindering further development of anatomical knowledge. Indeed, Galen's view of the circulatory system – that all vessels connected with the heart were arteries, while those connected with the liver were veins – dominated medicine for over a millennium. This was in part due to the prohibition on the

Drug history Enquire if the patient:

- has been treated previously for hypertension
- is currently taking any antihypertensive medication
- is intolerant to specific drugs previously prescribed for hypertension.
- is using drugs that can increase blood pressure (Table 1).

Table 1. Drugs that affect blood pressure.

Drugs that cause sodium retention

- Oral corticosteroids
- Adrenocorticotrophic hormone
- Carbenoxolone
- Nonsteroidal anti-inflammatory drugs

Drugs that cause increased sympathomimetic activity

- Ephedrine
- Cold cures
- Monoaminoxidase inhibitors

Direct vasoconstrictors

- Ergot alkaloids
- Combined oral contraceptives

Interactions with antihypertensive drugs

- Nonsteroidal anti-inflammatory drugs
- Tricyclic antidepressants

dissection of human cadavers, which was only lifted during the reign of Frederick II, Emperor of the Holy Roman Empire in 1220. Early in the 13th century, human dissection then became an important teaching tool at the University of Bologna, providing a firm base for understanding the structure and function of the cardiovascular system.

During the Renaissance, Leonardo da Vinci (1452–1519) dissected the human body and produced accurate descriptions and drawings

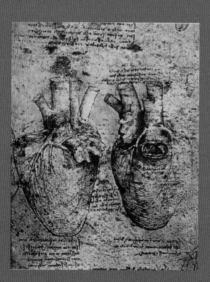

The heart – Leonardo da Vinci

of the heart and the coronary vasculature. Despite adhering to some of Galen's views – for instance, that blood passed between the ventricles through invisible pores in the septum – he was able to demonstrate that Galen had been wrong in believing that air entered the heart from the lungs. However,

Physical examination

General The physical examination should include a search for the causes and effects of hypertension and for the presence of other cardiovascular risk factors and of diseases that may affect the management strategy (Fig. 3).

Weight loss is often important for the control of blood pressure, so body weight should be recorded as a baseline for future measurements.

Secondary hypertension is very unusual but the clinical examination should aim to exclude secondary causes of hypertension, most of which are renal in origin (Table 2). When a remediable cause is identified, correction of that cause relieves the hypertension. Consider renovascular disease, renal disease, phaeochromocytoma and primary aldosteronism as possible causes of hypertension, if the patient has unusual symptoms such as :

- early age of onset
- abnormal renal function and electrolytes.

Table 2. Secondary causes of hypertension.

■ Diabetic nephropathy	■ Polycystic kidneys
■ Chronic pyelonephritis	■ Coarctation of the aorta
■ Obstructive uropathy	■ Phaeochromocytoma
■ Glomerulonephritis	■ Conn's syndrome
■ Renal artery stenosis	■ Cushing's syndrome

few knew of da Vinci's work until long after his death, as it was never published.

While earlier anatomists such as Mondino de Luzzi (1270–1326) from the University of Bologna had questioned Galen's invisible pores in the interventricular septum, it was with the publication in 1543 of *De Humani Corporis Fabrica* that Andreas Vesalius (1514–1564) laid the groundwork for observation-based

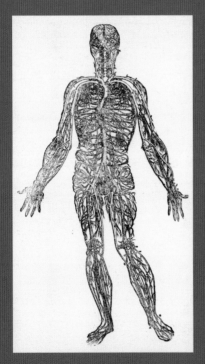

Circulatory system documented by Andreas Vesalius

anatomy. He took a more systematic approach to questioning Galen, where others had criticized only elements of Galen's views on anatomy while still adhering to some of Galen's more mystical notions.

Figure 3. Symptoms and signs of hypertension.

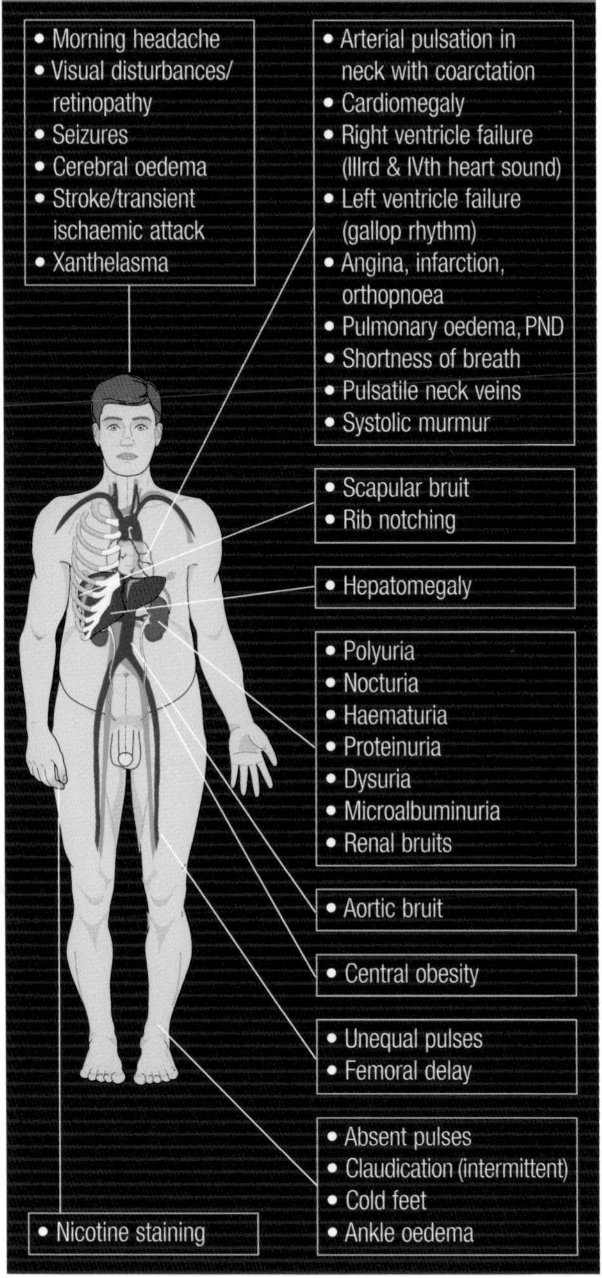

- Morning headache
- Visual disturbances/ retinopathy
- Seizures
- Cerebral oedema
- Stroke/transient ischaemic attack
- Xanthelasma

- Arterial pulsation in neck with coarctation
- Cardiomegaly
- Right ventricle failure (IIIrd & IVth heart sound)
- Left ventricle failure (gallop rhythm)
- Angina, infarction, orthopnoea
- Pulmonary oedema, PND
- Shortness of breath
- Pulsatile neck veins
- Systolic murmur

- Scapular bruit
- Rib notching

- Hepatomegaly

- Polyuria
- Nocturia
- Haematuria
- Proteinuria
- Dysuria
- Microalbuminuria
- Renal bruits

- Aortic bruit

- Central obesity

- Unequal pulses
- Femoral delay

- Absent pulses
- Claudication (intermittent)
- Cold feet
- Ankle oedema

- Nicotine staining

Vesalius produced anatomically exact descriptions of the human body based on dissection of human cadavers, noting that Galen had dissected only animals. He corrected many of Galen's 'observations' and poured scorn on the permeability of the septum. Perhaps more

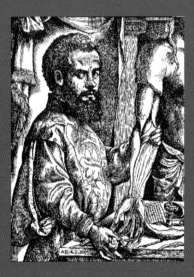

Anreas Vesalius dissecting the forearm of a corpse

importantly, he questioned why so many physicians and anatomists had followed Galen 'against reason'. Although this did not make him popular, it did mean that medicine would in the future focus on looking within bodies for the key to disease, rather than looking to external factors such as 'spirits'.

... completing the circuit

Even as late as the 16th century, it was still thought that blood ebbed and flowed to the

Measurement of blood pressure

Blood pressure should be measured on several occasions at intervals over a period of months.

- Choose a bladder and cuff size appropriate to the dimensions of the arm (Fig. 4)
- Ensure the patient is comfortably seated and rested for five minutes
- Support the arm at the level of the heart
- With mercury column measurement devices, place the manometer vertically, at eye level
- Estimate systolic pressure by palpating the brachial pulse and inflating the cuff until the pulsation disappears
- Inflate cuff to 30 mmHg above estimated systolic blood pressure
- Reduce manometer pressure at 2 mmHg per second during auscultation
- Take reading of diastolic blood pressure when repetitive sounds disappear
- Record pressures to the nearest 2 mmHg

Auscultatory sounds

- Phase 1 – The manometer reading at the point when repetitive, clear tapping sounds are heard for at least two consecutive beats is the systolic blood pressure
- Phase 5 – The manometer reading at which all sounds disappear completely is the diastolic blood pressure.

organs of the body, as described by Galen. But modern science and its achievements are founded upon observation and experiment, both of which gradually came to the fore.

Michael Servetus made the first published description of the pulmonary circulation in 1553. Further descriptions were published by Realdo Colombo in 1559 and by Andrea Cesalpino in 1571 and 1593. Although Cesalpino appears to have had an accurate view of the entire circulatory system, discovery of the circulatory system is generally accredited to the English physician William Harvey (1578–1657).

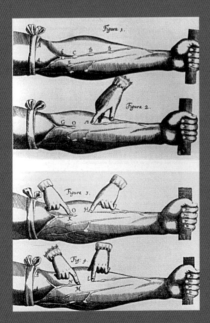

Figures 1 and 2 from William Harvey, Exercitatio Anatomica de Motu Cordus et Sanguinis in Animalibus, 1628, demonstrating the valves in the veins.

As a student in Padua, Harvey was exposed to the work of Servetus, Colombo and Cesalpino,

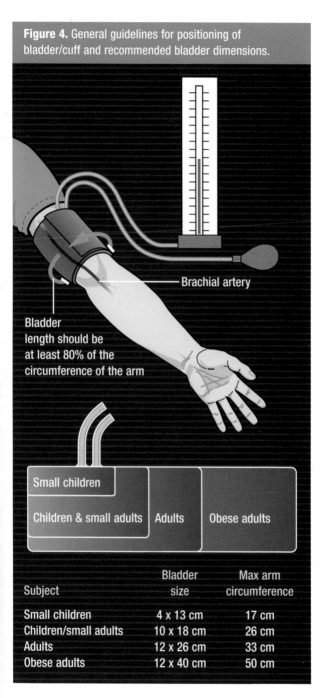

Figure 4. General guidelines for positioning of bladder/cuff and recommended bladder dimensions.

Brachial artery

Bladder length should be at least 80% of the circumference of the arm

Small children

Children & small adults   Adults   Obese adults

Subject	Bladder size	Max arm circumference
Small children	4 x 13 cm	17 cm
Children/small adults	10 x 18 cm	26 cm
Adults	12 x 26 cm	33 cm
Obese adults	12 x 40 cm	50 cm

19

and also studied with Fabrizio d'Acquapendente (1533–1619) who, in 1603, described the valves of the veins. This was a key discovery that fuelled Harvey's interest in the circulation. Through experimentation, he dispelled the myth of the ebb and flow of the blood with the publication of his classic work *Exercitatio Anatomica De Motu Cordis et Sanguinis in Animalibus* in 1628. He wrote that the purpose of the circulation was to transport life-giving blood to the tissues and then to return it to the heart where it could be re-nourished.

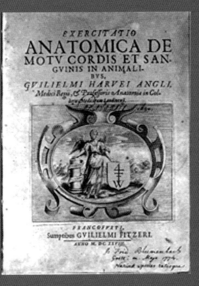

William Harvey, Exercitatio Anatomica de Motu Cordus et Sanguinis in Animalibus, 1628,

Importantly, Harvey based his notions on experimentation. He counted the number of heartbeats that occurred in a given time and showed that the volume of blood forced out of the heart in an hour far exceeded its volume in the whole animal, reasoning that the blood

Other general principles for accurate measurement of blood pressure are summarized in Table 3.

Table 3. General guidelines for blood pressure measurement

- Observe recommendations of national or international societies

- Measure routinely at least every 5 years in all adults until the age of 80 years

- Remeasure annually those with 'high–normal' values (135–139/85–89 mmHg)

- Make measurements in a consistent standardized fashion

- Measure sitting and standing in the elderly, diabetic or when symptoms indicate the need to detect postural hypotension

- Record both systolic and diastolic pressures

- Two or more readings separated by 2 minutes should be averaged; if the first two readings differ by more than 5 mmHg, additional readings should be taken

- Take readings at the same time of day relative to medication

- Note if the patient is anxious and this has affected blood pressure

- The presence of an auscultatory gap should be noted

- Maintain and service equipment regularly

- Calibrate automatic monitors regularly

must constantly move in a circuit, otherwise the arteries and body would explode under the pressure. Although he was able to show that a connection existed between the arteries and veins, he could not see the capillaries and so was unable to show the complete circulatory pathway. But he performed simple experiments using ligation to show that this connection existed, that the circulation was unidirectional, and that compression of the aorta led to dilation of the heart.

Direct observation of the linkage between arteries and veins was made possible by use of the newly invented light microscope. Although blood and air were previously thought to mingle freely in the lungs, Marcello Malpighi (1628–1694) used light microscopy to show the membraneous alveoli. He first wrote about the capillaries in 1661, thus completing the missing link in William Harvey's theory of the circulation.

... direct measurement of blood pressure

Harvey had proposed a closed circulatory system, making it clear that the blood in the arteries was under pressure. But there was no way of measuring that pressure until about one hundred years later. In 1733, the Reverend Stephen Hales (1677–1761) devised haemodynamic experiments and made the first direct measurement of blood pressure, which he described in *Haemastaticks* in 1733.

Other cardiovascular investigations

Pulses and bruits

- Auscultate the carotid and femoral pulses for bruits.
- Check the femoral pulse for volume and delay, which may suggest coarctation of the aorta or severe aortic arteriosclerosis.
- Examine the abdomen, with particular attention to the size of the liver and kidneys and the presence of a renal bruit – an insensitive sign – suggests renal artery stenosis.
- Palpation of the cardiac apex will identify gross left ventricular hypertrophy (LVH).

Sounds and cardiac murmurs

- The aortic component of the second heart sound is loud in the presence of raised blood pressure.
- A third heart sound or gallop rhythm may be heard if the left ventricle is failing.
- Basal crepitations during auscultation of the chest is suggestive of left ventricular failure.
- Look for indications of obstructive airways disease.
- Ejection systolic murmurs are common in hypertension. Consider the possibility of aortic valve disease particularly if a thrill is palpable, if the murmur is of high grade, or if the aortic component of the second heart sound is quiet (suggestive of aortic stenosis).

Hales – the father of sphygmomanometry – inserted a brass tube into the jugular vein and carotid artery of a horse and connected this to a vertical glass tube containing water, allowing him to measure blood pressure in feet and inches. He showed that arterial pressure was greater than venous pressure and reasoned that peak blood pressure occurred when the heart contracted, thus representing cardiac output, while the lowest level of blood pressure occurred when the heart was relaxed, representing resistance to flow.

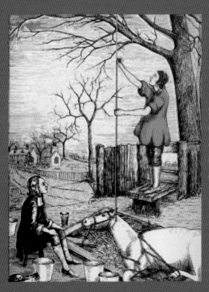

Stephen Hales' experiment to determine the blood pressure of a horse

A century later, in 1828, Jean-Leonard Marie Poiseuille accurately measured blood pressure in animals using a mercury manometer connected to a cannula inserted directly into an artery.

- Coarctation of the aorta may be associated with a loud systolic murmur over the left precordium with radiation into the left scapular region, where pulsation may be palpable.
- Coarctation rarely causes symptoms but may present with claudication.

The eyes

- Examination of the optic fundi should be an integral part of the assessment.
- Ophthalmoscopy rapidly identifies those patients with severe and malignant hypertension and is particularly helpful in the assessment of older patients, in whom it can reveal visual impairment caused by hypertension.

Additional investigations

The British Hypertension Society (BHS) recommends five routine investigations.

- Urine strip test for blood and protein
- Serum creatinine and electrolytes
- Blood glucose
- Serum total:high-density lipoprotein (HDL) cholesterol
- Electrocardiogram (ECG)

Haematuria may occur in patients with malignant hypertension and glomerular diseases,

Using Poiseuille's manometer, the French physician Jean Faivre made the first direct intra-arterial measurement of blood pressure in humans; clearly less invasive approaches were required before blood pressure measurement would have any practical use.

Karl Vierodt (1818–1884) introduced the sphygmograph for indirect measurement of blood pressure in 1854 with the development of a cumbersome and somewhat inaccurate device that measured the amount of pressure needed to obliterate the radial pulse. This idea was refined by the French physiologist Etienne Jules Marey (1830–1904), who developed a sphygmograph by which the radial pulse wave was transmitted directly to a metal plate applied closely to the skin of the forearm and amplified mechanically before being recorded on smoked paper. Although it was useful for recording blood pressure and cardiac rhythm, this device proved rather too unwieldy for everyday use.

Samuel Siegfried von Basch, a physician in Vienna, developed the first non-invasive sphygmomanometer in 1881 using an inflatable rubber bag with water, and also established a normal range of systolic blood pressure, which he considered to be around 150 mmHg. This device was introduced into hospital practice.

But it was in 1896 that Scipione Riva-Rocci (1863–1920) developed the prototype of the instrument still in use today. His device used an

but may occur with bladder neoplasia, which must be excluded. Proteinuria is commonplace, especially in malignant hypertension and in patients with underlying renal disease. An ECG may provide evidence of LVH which increases the total cardiovascular risk. It may also show undetected arrhythmias and evidence of previous MI or ischaemia. When the ECG shows a 'high' left ventricular voltage without T-wave abnormalities (often the case in young patients) an echocardiogram is useful to confirm a diagnosis of LVH, the degree of hypertrophy and to monitor the response to treatment.

The clinical history may indicate the need for additional tests, including:

- full blood count if there are indications of alcohol over-consumption or abuse.
- uric acid if there is a history of gout or renal disease.
- urinalysis for catecholamines if the history suggests phaechromocytoma.
- ultrasound examination of the kidneys or intravenous pyelography if renal disease is suspected.

Interpretations of blood tests are summarised in Table 4. Refer the patient to a specialist if the investigations suggest a need for further tests or if the patient is young.

inflatable rubber bag encased in a non-expandable cuff. Inflation of the cuff by means of an attached rubber bulb would compress the

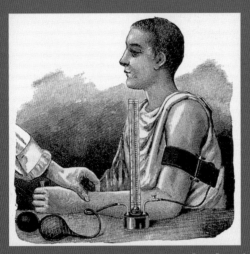

Riva-Rocca's sphygmomanometer in use (1908)

arm until it occluded the brachial artery, and a mercury manometer registered the pressure within the cuff. The appearance of oscillations in the column of mercury coincided with the reappearance of the radial pulse by palpation as the rubber bag was deflated. At this point the cuff pressure was equal to the arterial pulse and the level of the mercury column gave the systolic pressure.

Despite providing no measure of diastolic pressure, Riva-Rocci's sphygmomanometer represents a major milestone in the history of hypertension, and it soon passed into

Complementary questions to consider are:

- what is the level of blood pressure?
- has the high blood pressure caused target organ damage?
- are there associated cardiovascular risk factors?

Some of the factors that influence overall risk are summarised in Table 5.

Table 5. Risk factors for cardiovascular diseases

Modifiable:

- High LDL cholesterol
- High blood pressure
- Smoking
- Low HDL cholesterol
- Lack of exercise
- Diabetes (± glucose intolerance) especially with proteinuria
- Left ventricular hypertrophy
- Central obesity
- Clotting factors
- Oral contraceptives
- Sedentary lifestyle

Non-modifiable:

- Age
- Sex
- Family history
- Genetics
- Birth weight

vasoconstriction. Like Bernard, Brown-Séquard also worked on the endocrine functions of the kidney, and his work effectively set the stage for the discovery of renin.

Physicians working at this time began to view physical examination of the patient as crucial, and began to relate findings in life with pathological changes seen at post-mortem, observations that would, in time, allow them to make the crucial link between blood pressure and disease.

Richard Bright (1789–1858), a physician at Guy's Hospital, London, noted in 1836 that patients with chronic renal disease ('albuminous urine') often showed hypertrophy of the left

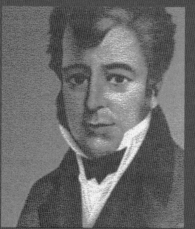

Richard Bright
(1789–1858)

ventricle, and suggested that this may have been a consequence of an altered quality of the blood or the increased force needed to drive blood through diseased vasculature.

Associated clinical conditions, including target organ damage:

Cerebrovascular disease

- Ischaemic stroke
- Cerebral haemorrhage
- Transient ischaemic attack

Heart disease

- Myocardial infarction
- Angina
- Coronary revascularization
- Congestive heart failure
- Left ventricular hypertrophy

Renal disease

- Diabetic nephropathy
- Renal impairment – plasma creatinine concentration >1.2 mg/dl
- Proteinuria

Peripheral arterial disease

- Abdominal aortic aneurysm
- Intermittent claudication

Advanced hypertensive retinopathy

- Haemorrhages or exudates
- Papilloedema

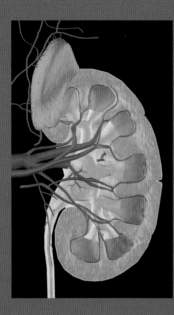

The condition he described – nephritis and albuminuria, usually accompanied by oedema and elevated blood pressure – came to be known as Bright's disease. Although Bright did not make the explicit link with hypertension, subsequent physicians such as George Johnson in 1868 mentioned increased peripheral resistance as the basis for left ventricular hypertrophy and correlated this with elevated arterial pressure.

In his microscopic studies, the Victorian physician Sir William Withey Gull (1816–1891) also focused attention on the broader vascular system. He believed that the cardiac effects of Bright's disease were due not to renal failure but to changes in the entire capillary system, and showed in 1872 that the walls of smaller arteries were thickened even in patients who showed no evidence of renal disease. However, he suggested that these pathological changes were due to a primary disease of the blood vessels rather than to high blood pressure.

Figure 5 illustrates how these associated clinical conditions and target organ damage can be integrated into a treatment algorithm for patients with different levels of blood pressure. To calculate the 10 year CHD risk several methods are available. The most accurate chart method currently recorded in the UK is the *Joint British Societies Coronary Risk Prediction Charts* for primary prevention. See pages 39-49.

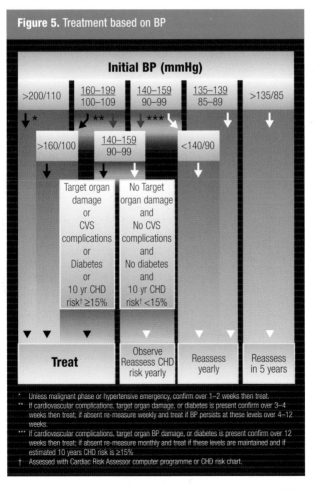

Figure 5. Treatment based on BP

* Unless malignant phase or hypertensive emergency, confirm over 1–2 weeks then treat.
** If cardiovascular complications, target organ damage, or diabetes is present confirm over 3–4 weeks then treat; if absent re-measure weekly and treat if BP persists at these levels over 4–12 weeks.
*** If cardiovascular complications, target organ BP damage, or diabetes is present confirm over 12 weeks then treat; if absent re-measure monthly and treat if these levels are maintained and if estimated 10 years CHD risk is ≥15%
† Assessed with Cardiac Risk Assessor computer programme or CHD risk chart.

The neurologist Sir William Richard Gowers (1845–1915), who pioneered the use of the ophthalmoscope, showed a correlation between

Constriction of arterioles in the retina.

raised arterial pressure and constriction of arterioles in the retina. He was also able to demonstrate vascular changes in the retina of patients with Bright's disease.

Frederick Mahomed (1849–1884) was one of the first physicians to measure blood pressure as part of his routine clinical evaluation of patients, using his own modified sphygmograph based on that of Etienne Jules Marey. In 1874, in his paper entitled *The Etiology of Bright's Disease and the Prealbuminuric Stage*, Mahomed noted that acute nephritis was associated with increased arterial pressure. Importantly, he also recognized the existence of high blood pressure without obvious cause and in the absence of albuminuria. Albutt confirmed this in 1895, and coined the term 'hyperpiesia' for patients with elevated blood pressure without Bright's disease. Subsequently, hyperpiesia came to be known as essential hypertension and knowledge of its natural history began to be pieced together.

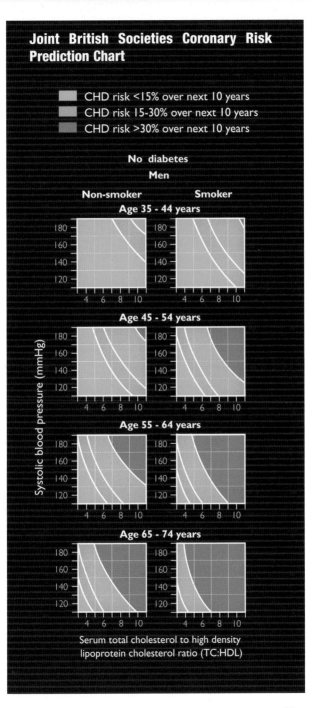

Joint British Societies Coronary Risk Prediction Chart

- CHD risk <15% over next 10 years
- CHD risk 15-30% over next 10 years
- CHD risk >30% over next 10 years

No diabetes

Men

Non-smoker   **Smoker**

Age 35 - 44 years

Age 45 - 54 years

Age 55 - 64 years

Age 65 - 74 years

Systolic blood pressure (mmHg)

Serum total cholesterol to high density lipoprotein cholesterol ratio (TC:HDL)

Theodore Janeway at Columbia University began recording his observations on systolic blood pressure using Riva-Rocci's sphygmomanometer in 1903, before adopting Korotkoff's auscultatory method a few years later. Janeway clearly recognized that hypertension, which he regarded as a blood pressure level above 160 mmHg, was primarily a vascular rather than a renal disease.

Hypertension… causes, effects and treatments

Throughout the 20th century, a number of theories have been proposed as the cause of hypertension. At various times it has been considered a disease of renal or adrenal origin, the consequence of abnormal salt balance, disturbance of the sympathetic nervous system and so on. Similarly, fashionable ideas on treatment have included, at various times, haemodynamic, endocrinological and even surgical approaches.

In 1949, Irwin Page at the Rockefeller Institute developed what he called the mosaic theory of hypertension, challenging the prevailing assumption that hypertension was due to a single cause. Page argued that the function of blood pressure was to distribute blood throughout the whole body and that the body had a variety of mechanisms to regulate this function.

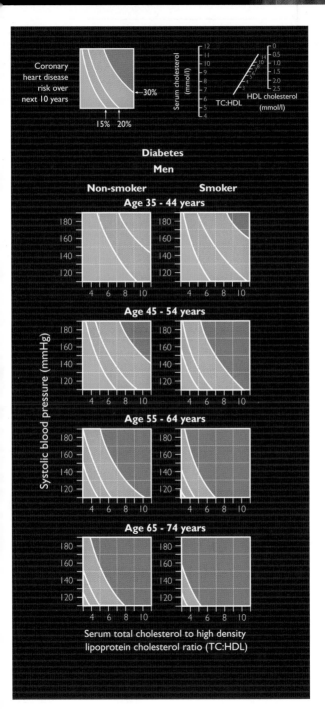

Coronary heart disease risk over next 10 years

15% 20% 30%

Serum cholesterol (mmol/l)

TC:HDL   HDL cholesterol (mmol/l)

Diabetes

Men

Non-smoker **Smoker**

Age 35 - 44 years

Age 45 - 54 years

Systolic blood pressure (mmHg)

Age 55 - 64 years

Age 65 - 74 years

Serum total cholesterol to high density lipoprotein cholesterol ratio (TC:HDL)

41

Even today, much is still unknown about the pathophysiology of essential hypertension. While an underlying renal or adrenal disease is the cause of raised blood pressure in a small number of patients (2–5%), in the remainder there is no clear, identifiable cause. Nevertheless, as scientific work has progressed it has become increasingly clear that hypertension is a multifactorial disorder. A number of physiological mechanisms have been shown to be involved in the maintenance of blood pressure; derangement of any may play a part in the development of hypertension. Each, therefore, represents a potential therapeutic target.

... neural and humoral mechanisms

Elucidation of the role of humoral substances in the vasomotor control of hypertension began in 1894, when an adrenal gland extract isolated by Oliver and Schäfer was shown to result in marked increases in blood pressure. Subsequently, this was shown to lead to an increase in peripheral resistance through arteriolar constriction. The active component – adrenaline – was shown by the Cambridge physiologist Thomas Elliott in 1905 to have the same activity in any part of the body as stimulation of the sympathetic nerves serving that part of the body. He proposed that the neurotransmitter involved in sympathetic stimulation was adrenaline or a substance related to it.

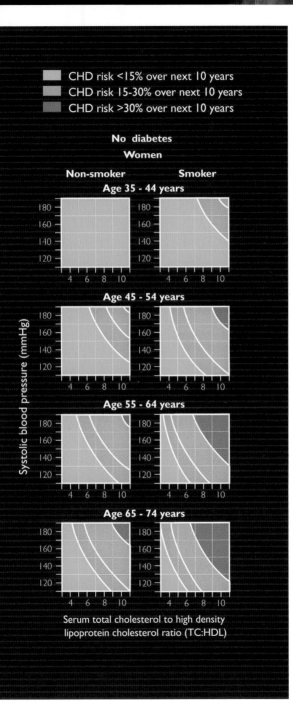

CHD risk <15% over next 10 years
CHD risk 15-30% over next 10 years
CHD risk >30% over next 10 years

No diabetes
Women

Non-smoker   **Smoker**

Age 35 - 44 years

Age 45 - 54 years

Age 55 - 64 years

Age 65 - 74 years

Systolic blood pressure (mmHg)

Serum total cholesterol to high density
lipoprotein cholesterol ratio (TC:HDL)

Experiments by Sir Henry Dale at Cambridge and Otto Loewi in Graz demonstrated that acetylcholine is released from parasympathetic nerve endings and is responsible for vasodilatation. Loewi and Dale shared the Nobel Prize in 1936 for their work on the chemical control of nerve impulses, which had paved the way to understanding of the control of the autonomic nervous system and its contribution to blood pressure control.

The earliest antihypertensive agents targeted vasomotor control through the neural mechanisms elucidated by these physiologists: these included veratrum alkaloids, thiocyanates, the ganglion-blockers and the centrally acting antihypertensives. Despite lowering blood pressure, many of these agents were poorly tolerated or had unacceptable side effects.

The centrally acting antihypertensives were among the first safe and effective agents and were introduced in the 1950s. They act centrally, by reducing sympathetic drive, which is responsible for maintaining cardiac output, arterial tone and body fluid volume. However, because of their central side effects, they can only be used in low doses. Current centrally acting antihypertensives such as reserpine, clonidine and methyldopa are generally used only as second- or third-line treatment.

Ambard and Beaujard demonstrated the hypertensive effect of salt in 1904, and some doctors subsequently adopted dietary salt

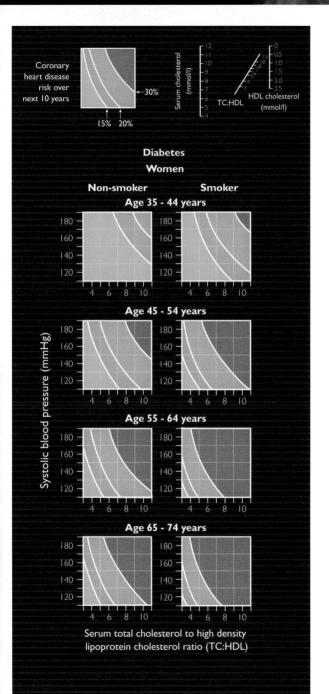

Coronary heart disease risk over next 10 years

30%

15% 20%

Serum cholesterol (mmol/l)

TC:HDL

HDL cholesterol (mmol/l)

Diabetes

Women

Non-smoker   **Smoker**

Age 35 - 44 years

Age 45 - 54 years

Systolic blood pressure (mmHg)

Age 55 - 64 years

Age 65 - 74 years

Serum total cholesterol to high density lipoprotein cholesterol ratio (TC:HDL)

45

restriction as a means of lowering high blood pressure. However, a more effective means of reducing blood volume became available in the 1950s with the development of the thiazide diuretics.

The earliest diuretics were organomercurial agents. Although they lowered blood pressure, they required parenteral administration and were associated with unacceptable toxicity. The development of orally active thiazide diuretics

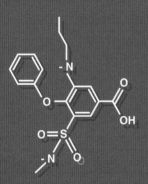

Bumetanide – a loop diuretic introduced in the 1960s

such as chlorothiazide and hydrochlorothiazide, which inhibit sodium reabsorption at the distal convoluted tubule within the kidney, made it possible to reduce oedema and thus blood pressure. Loop diuretics such as frusemide and bumetanide were introduced in the 1960s. Despite being powerful diuretics, they were found to promote hypokalaemia, so potassium-sparing diuretics such as amiloride and spironolactone were developed.

Diuretics remain in widespread use for the treatment of hypertension. However, they are

How to use the Coronary Risk Prediction Chart for Primary Prevention

These charts are for estimating coronary heart disease (CHD) risk (non-fatal MI, coronary death and new angina pectoris) for individuals who have not already developed CHD or other major atherosclerotic disease. They are an aid to making clinical decisions about how intensively to intervene on lifestyle and whether to use antihypertensive and lipid lowering medication, but should **not replace clinical judgment**.

The use of these charts is not appropriate for patients who have existing diseases which already put them at high risk. Such diseases are:

– CHD or other major atherosclerotic disease

– Familial hypercholesterolaemia or other inherited dyslipidaemias

– Renal dysfunction including diabetic nephropathy

■ The charts should also not be used to decide whether to introduce antihypertensive medication when blood pressure persistently exceeds 160/100 or when target organ damage due to hypertension is present. In both cases antihypertensive medication is recommended regardless of CHD risk.

■ To estimate an individual's absolute 10 year risk of developing CHD choose the table for his or her gender, diabetes (yes/no), smoking status (smoker/non-smoker) and age. Within this square define the level of risk according to the point where the coordinates for systolic blood pressure and the ratio of total cholesterol to high density lipoprotein (HDL) cholesterol meet. If no HDL cholesterol result is available, then assume this is 1.00mmol/l and the lipid scale can be used for total serum cholesterol alone. Diabetes refers to type 2 diabetes. See later note, if patient has type 1 diabetes or impaired fasting glucose.

■ High risk individuals are defined as those whose 10 year CHD risk exceeds 15% equivalent to a combined risk of CHD and stroke (cardiovascular risk) of >20% over the same period. As a minimum those at highest CHD risk (>30% red) should be targeted and treated now, and as resources allow others with a CHD risk of >15% (orange) should be progressively targeted.

■ Smoking status should reflect lifetime exposure to tobacco and not simply tobacco use at the time of assessment e.g. those who have given up smoking within 5 years may be regarded as current smokers. Ex-smokers with prolonged or heavy exposure more than 5 years ago may continue to be at higher risk than life-long non-smokers.

continued on page 49

associated with side effects such as polyuria and impotence, and at high doses they can induce electrolyte disturbances as well as alterations in lipid metabolism and glucose tolerance, limitations which have led researchers to continue the search for alternative means of lowering blood pressure.

In 1948, Ahlquist explained the fact that adrenaline would both excite and inhibit smooth muscle by suggesting that catecholamine activity was mediated by alpha and beta receptors. Alpha-adrenoceptors mediated excitatory functions and beta-adrenoceptors mediated inhibitory functions, except in the heart, where excitatory adrenoceptors were mainly of the alpha type. The subsequent search for agents that could block these receptors, and thus neutralize the effects of catecholamines, led to the discovery of **beta-blockers** and later **alpha-blockers**.

The first beta-blocker was synthesized in 1958, but was found to have partial agonist activity, making it unsuitable for clinical use. In 1962, Black and Stephenson described propranolol, a competitive beta-adrenergic antagonist free from agonist activity, which was shown to have antihypertensive activity as well as anti-anginal activity.

Subsequently, identification of beta-1 receptors localized in the heart and beta-2 receptors localized in other smooth muscle cells has led to the development of a range of beta-blockers

continued from page 47

■ The initial blood pressure and the first random (non-fasting) total cholesterol and HDL cholesterol can be used to estimate an individual's risk. However, the decision on using drug therapy should generally be based on repeat risk factor measurements over a period of time.

■ These charts (and all other currently available methods of CHD risk prediction) are based on groups of people with untreated levels of blood pressure, total cholesterol and HDL cholesterol. In patients already receiving antihypertensive therapy in whom the decision is to be made about whether to introduce lipid-lowering medication or vice versa the charts can act as a guide, but unless recent pre-treatment risk factor values are available it is generally safest to assume that CHD risk is higher than that predicted by current levels of blood pressure or lipids on treatment.

■ CHD risk is also higher than indicated in the charts for:

  – Those with a family history of premature CHD (male first degree relatives aged <55 years and female first degree relatives aged <65 years) which increases the risk by a factor of approximately 1.5

  – Those with raised triglyceride levels

  – Women with premature menopause

  – Those who are not yet diabetic but have impaired fasting glucose (6.1-6.9mmol.l)

  – Patients with Type 1 diabetes in whom the risk is often greater than predicted by the total cholesterol to HDL cholesterol ratio. It may be more accurate to ignore HDL cholesterol in them and use the lipid scale for total serum cholesterol alone, but direct evidence for this is currently lacking.

  – As the person approaches the next age category. As risk increases exponentially with age the risk will be closer to the higher decennium for the last four years of each decade.

■ In ethnic minorities the risk charts should be used with caution because they have not been validated in these populations e.g. in people originating from the Indian subcontinent it is safest to assume that the CHD risk is higher than predicted from the charts.

■ An individual can be shown on the chart the direction in which his or her risk of CHD can be reduced by changing smoking status, blood pressure or cholesterol, but it should be borne in mind that the estimate of risk is for a group of people with similar risk factors and that within that group there will be considerable variation in risk. The charts are primarily to assist in directing intervention to those who statistically stand to benefit most.

that differ in relative affinity for these receptors and so differ in the effects and side effects. More recently, beta-3 receptors have been characterized.

Because they have been shown to be highly effective antihypertensive agents associated with reduced mortality and morbidity from both coronary heart disease and stroke, beta-blockers are still widely used in the treatment of hypertension, as well as for patients with ischaemic heart disease and certain arrythmias. In recognition of his achievement in developing the first beta-blocker, in 1988, Sir James Black was awarded the Nobel Prize.

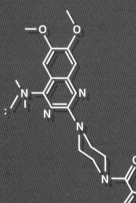

Selective alpha-1-adrenoceptor antagonists, prazosin

Since Smithwick showed in the 1950s that sympathectomy resulted in lowering of elevated blood pressure, increased sympathetic nervous system activity has been thought to be important in initiating and maintaining

Initial treatment measures All patients should be given advice on diet and lifestyle measures for the control of hypertension and/or reduction of overall cardiovascular risk (Table 6). In favourable circumstances non-drug measures can lower blood pressure as much as drug monotherapy and in some cases may eliminate the need for drug treatment. When drug treatment is necessary lifestyle changes measures may:

- enhance the antihypertensive effect of drugs
- reduce the need for polypharmacy.

Table 6. Lifestyle measures to reduce blood pressure and cardiovascular risk.

Measures that reduce blood pressure
Weight reduction
Reduce salt intake
Limit alcohol consumption
Physical exercise
Increase fruit and vegetable consumption
Reduce total fat and saturated fat intake

Measures to reduce cardiovascular risk
Stop smoking
Replace saturated fat with polyunsaturated fat and mono-unsaturated fats
Increase oily fish consumption
Reduce total fat intake

hypertension. This led to the development of drugs that lower sympathetic tone, and thus hypertension, by acting at sympathetic nerve endings. Many early drugs such as the ganglion blockers and the non-selective alpha-adrenoceptor antagonists, were found to have unacceptable side effects and are no longer used. However, selective alpha-1-adrenoceptor antagonists such as prazosin, terazosin and doxazosin are now widely used in the treatment of hypertension.

... the renin-angiotensin-aldosterone system

Although Bright and his successors had made the link between hypertension and the kidney, it was in 1894 that Robert Tigerstedt first described a substance formed in the kidneys that could under normal conditions pass into the blood stream via internal secretion and exert a hypertensive effect. They had discovered renin, and for several years it was thought that the kidney might be responsible for hypertension. Subsequently, Harry Goldblatt in 1934 induced hypertension in dogs by constricting one renal artery and reversed it by removal of the clamp, a procedure shown in 1940 to stimulate renin production by the ischaemic kidney.

Around the same time, various groups around the world elucidated the elements of the renin-angiotensin system. Renin was shown to act on

Weight

Encouraging patients to loose weight can have a very favourable effect on blood pressure. The application of simple general principles can be highly effective.

- Advice should be given in positive terms, not as a series of orders or prohibitions.
- The diet should be discussed in the context of the whole family and should involve a review of cooking methods and shopping habits.
- Reducing fat consumption is a highly effective method of losing weight. It also lowers cholesterol levels.
- Reduction in salt intake is advisable (see next section). This may mean examining and reducing the consumption of prepared foods, many of which have a high salt content.
- Fresh fruit and vegetables are filling and usually low in calories. They are also a rich source of vitamins, anti-oxidants, complex carbohydrates and some dietary fibre. For all these reasons their consumption should be strongly encouraged.
- Eating large meals late at night should be discouraged as this promotes weight gain.
- Weight should be lost gradually over a prolonged period. Patients are likely to need encouragement during this time, so it is important to be committed and enthusiastic, and to provide clear well-informed advice.

a plasma protein (later identified as angiotensinogen) to form a substance (initially called hypertensin, later called angiotensin) that raises blood pressure.

In the 1950s, simultaneous work by groups in Cleveland, USA, and at St Mary's Hospital, London, resulted in isolation of two forms of angiotensin: the active compound angiotensin II was shown to be formed from the enzymatic conversion of angiotensin I catalysed by angiotensin converting enzyme. Angiotensin II has been shown to be the most powerful pressor agent known: in the 1970s, it was shown that angiotensin II actually harms the heart and kidney and that patients with high levels of plasma-renin activity are at increased risk of stroke or myocardial infarction.

Also in the 1950s, work began to reveal the physiological role of aldosterone in the hormonal control of blood pressure, which is also controlled by angiotensin II. Subsequently, it has been shown that sustained elevation of blood pressure requires interplay between renin-angiotensin and aldosterone.

Further work on renin by Harry Goldblatt and John Laragh's group at Cornell prompted the development of pharmacological agents able to block the renin-angiotensin-aldosterone system.

The concept of treating hypertension by blockade of the renin-angiotensin system was established in the 1970s with the development

Sodium and potassium

A reduction in sodium intake of 100 mmol is associated with an approximately 6 mmHg reduction in systolic blood pressure. The effect of salt restriction is greater in older patients. Combination of salt restriction with drug therapy usually produces a greater blood pressure reduction than drugs alone, although calcium antagonists appear to be an exception to this general rule.

Helping patients to reduce dietary salt intake requires detailed advice because sodium is found in very high quantities in many staple foods – for example bread. Patients need to be encouraged to reduce their use of prepared and canned foods, many of which are high in salt. Salted nuts are another common source of dietary salt.

An increase in dietary potassium intake may be appropriate for many patients. A 100mmol/L increase in the intake of potassium is associated with an approximately 10mmHg reduction in systolic blood pressure. Some of the best sources of dietary potassium are fruits and vegetables; increased consumption of these will normally be recommended as part of general lifestyle and weight reduction measures. Dried figs, mushrooms, bananas and orange juice all contain large amounts of potassium.

> High-potassium diets are contraindicated in patients with impaired renal function, or renal failure.

of saralasin, an antagonist of the angiotensin II receptor. Although this agent lowered blood pressure and improved haemodynamics in congestive heart failure, the need for intravenous administration limited its utility. In addition, at higher doses, partial agonist effects emerged.

Sergio Ferreira first identified angiotensin converting enzyme (ACE) inhibitors in 1965; he isolated peptides in snake venom able to potentiate the activity of bradykinin, a potent

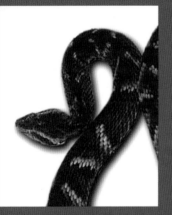

Sergio Ferreira isolated peptides in snake venom are able to potentiate the activity of bradykinin.

vasodilator. Others showed that these peptides blocked the conversion of angiotensin I to angiotensin II, leading directly to the synthesis of captopril, the first orally active ACE inhibitor for the treatment of hypertension, in the late 1970s. This and the agents that followed have helped to define the contribution of the renin-angiotensin-aldosterone system to the control of blood pressure. Today, blockade of the renin-angiotensin system by ACE inhibitors such as

Alcohol consumption

Alcohol appears to increase blood pressure. 'Binge' drinking, whereby most of the week's alcohol intake is concentrated into one or two nights may be more harmful than drinking moderate amounts of alcohol most nights of the week. In any event, excessive alcohol consumption should be discouraged. For patients with hypertension, the number of units of alcohol (Fig. 6) should be restricted to 21/week for men and 14/week for women.

Simple measures can be suggested to help people whose social activities emphasize drinking.

- Change the type of beer or lager drunk to a brand containing less alcohol.
- Add soda water to wine.

Figure 6. The maximum recommended intake of alcohol is 21 units/week for men and 14 units/week for women.

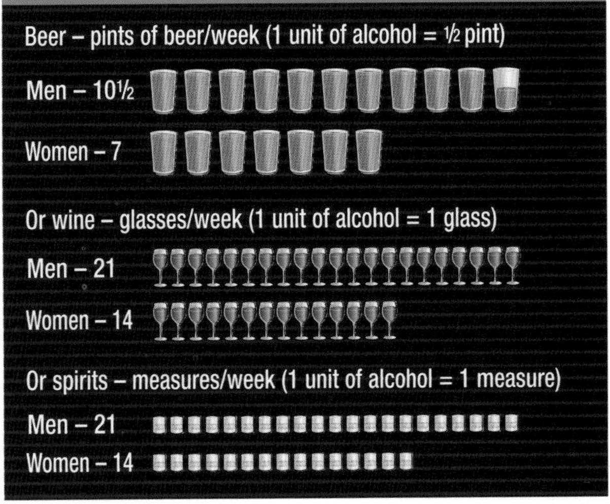

Beer – pints of beer/week (1 unit of alcohol = ½ pint)
Men – 10½
Women – 7

Or wine – glasses/week (1 unit of alcohol = 1 glass)
Men – 21
Women – 14

Or spirits – measures/week (1 unit of alcohol = 1 measure)
Men – 21
Women – 14

enalapril, lisinopril, trandolapril and perindopril is an important contributor to the control of hypertension and the reduction in morbidity and mortality from congestive heart failure.

In addition, ACE inhibitors have been shown to reduce proteinuria, making them valuable agents in the treatment of chronic renal disease.

However, because ACE is not specific for angiotensin I and also catalyses the inactivation of bradykinin, ACE inhibition results in build up of bradykinin levels (as Ferreira noted), which are responsible for the most frequent side effects of ACE inhibitors (cough and angio-oedema). With the development of non-peptide, orally active angiotensin II receptor antagonists such as losartan, candesartan, valsartan, irbesartan and telmisartan, it has become possible to block the renin-angiotensin system without raising bradykinin levels.

... the role of calcium in vasodilatation

Calcium has been known to play an important role in the regulation of cellular processes since Sidney Ringer (1835–1910) at University College London noticed that it was required for contraction of isolated myocardial tissue. But it was in the later part of the 20th century that its role in arterial contraction, and thus peripheral resistance, was recognized.

Physical exercise

Regular aerobic exercise has a moderate blood pressure-lowering effect. The benefits of exercise on overall cardiovascular risk extend beyond blood pressure, however, and include improved lipid profile and insulin resistance.

Exercise should be regular, but does not need to be vigorous. In general, activity should be increased gradually and should be repeated at least three times weekly for about 30 minutes each session. The preferred form of exercise is aerobic (e.g., walking, swimming, and cycling) rather than isometric (such as weight lifting). In an essentially sedentary society, even minimal increases in activity confer benefits (Fig 7). Brisk walking is sufficient to provide cardiovascular training in a majority of people.

Advice on exercises must be practical and realistic, tailored to the medical and social conditions of the patient – if exercise cannot be taken in a manner that is convenient and agreeable to the patient it is unlikely to be maintained long-term. For example, swimming is an excellent option for patients, particularly older people, whose capacity for weight-bearing exercise is limited by osteoarthritis and other musculo-skeletal infirmities. Dancing is a unique combination of exercise and socializing and should be encouraged in patients who enjoy it. Sports and leisure centres increasingly run fitness and training programmes appropriate to

In 1964, Albrecht Fleckenstein reported that two new synthetic vasodilator compounds, later named verapamil and prenylamine, mimicked the effects of calcium deficiency on heart muscle: essentially, they depressed the myocardium. Since restoring the calcium supply to the contractile system neutralized this effect, he called the agents calcium antagonists.

Subsequently, a large number of other calcium antagonists were synthesized. Further studies showed that they selectively inhibited the slow movement of calcium ions into the slow channels of active cell membranes within the myocardial fibres, and the drugs were renamed **calcium-channel blockers**.

With his co-workers, Fleckenstein showed that contraction of all smooth muscle cells is dependent on the inward flux of calcium ions, and that calcium overload in the heart muscle leads to necrosis of fibres, which can be prevented in the presence of a calcium-channel blocker. Initially, these agents were marketed for the management of ischaemic heart disease; today, because they decrease blood pressure through their arterial dilating properties, they are recognized as a major class of antihypertensive agent.

Subsequently, calcium-channel blockers have been shown to be a heterogeneous group of drugs. Older agents such as verapamil and diltiazem will slow atrioventricular conduction and are negatively inotropic; the newer

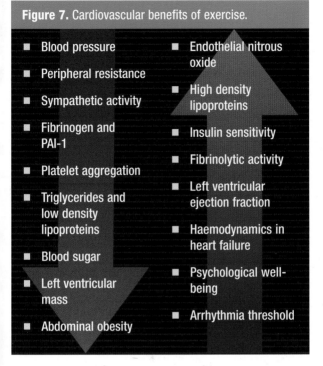

Figure 7. Cardiovascular benefits of exercise.

- Blood pressure
- Peripheral resistance
- Sympathetic activity
- Fibrinogen and PAI-1
- Platelet aggregation
- Triglycerides and low density lipoproteins
- Blood sugar
- Left ventricular mass
- Abdominal obesity

- Endothelial nitrous oxide
- High density lipoproteins
- Insulin sensitivity
- Fibrinolytic activity
- Left ventricular ejection fraction
- Haemodynamics in heart failure
- Psychological well-being
- Arrhythmia threshold

different age groups and this too can add a social dimension that is an important source of motivation for many people.

In some instances it may be necessary to caution patients against excessive enthusiasm for exercise. A sudden change from inactivity to strenuous exercising involves some risks, not all of them cardiovascular. Such patients are, however, relatively rare.

The value of exercise as part of cardiac rehabilitation schemes has been proved. A history past MI is in itself no obstacle to a patient implementing an exercise plan.

subgroup of dihydropyridine calcium-channel blockers such as amlodipine, felodipine, nifedipine, nicardipine, nisoldipine, lercanidipine and lacidipine are non-rate limiting and have a more selective action on vascular tissue. Recent research suggests that these newer agents reduce the risk of end-organ disease such as left ventricular hypertrophy, renal disease, and even atherosclerosis.

Epidemiology as a research tool

Although laboratory work is undoubtedly important to the development of medical science, one reason why understanding and management of hypertension have progressed so far in recent decades has been the ability to gather information on the natural history of cardiovascular disease through population-level research.

The earliest epidemiological work on hypertension was conducted by life insurance companies, whose doctors had noted that people with high blood pressure died at a younger age than those with normal blood pressure.

As far back as the 18th century, life insurance companies began to calculate premiums on the basis of actuarial data, or life tables, based on expected mortality within the population. In the 19th century, insurance companies began to

Smoking The health benefits of stopping smoking are huge and extend far beyond hypertension. The fact that there are great benefits to be obtained from not smoking does not, however, mean that it is easy to stop.

Constructive advice to patients on how to stop smoking must recognize the powerful addictive property of nicotine and the integration of smoking habits as part of daily routines. Combining clear advice about the risks of smoking and the benefits of stopping with a recognition that many people would have stopped smoking of their own accord if it was easy to do so helps create a useful rapport with the patient. Most people who finally succeed in giving up smoking have tried and failed on several previous occasions; support and encouragement for those who relapse is a logical and humane attitude. Health professionals themselves should be encouraged by the evidence that their advice is a powerful influence. One of the most common explanations offered by ex-smokers of why they gave up is that their physician told them to. The power of example is also immense; any physician who advises patients to stop smoking while himself continuing to smoke is unlikely to be taken seriously.

Effective 'stop smoking' plans combine a strategy for gradual nicotine withdrawal, together with behaviour modification designed take into account the medical background of those seeking insurance, usually based on their environmental risk of contracting contagious diseases. By the end of the 19th century, the insurance companies were collecting information using detailed medical questionnaires and medical examinations conducted by highly qualified physicians for prognostic information on their clients. By 1875, the sphygmograph was being used in

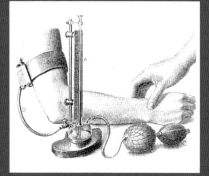

By 1875, the sphygmograph was being used in medical examinations by insurance companies.

medical examinations by certain insurance companies, and was used to study 'generalized arteriosclerosis' and the loss of arterial compliance that was often noted at autopsy. By 1899, they would also routinely look for albuminuria, as evidence of Bright's disease. Thus, even before hypertension was fully understood and existed as a medical concept, the insurance companies accepted the idea of 'vascular risk'.

Subsequently, with the availability of instruments for measuring blood pressure, the American insurance companies promoted the use of the

to break, in a positive way, the association of particular events with cigarette smoking. The number of cigarettes and their nicotine content should be gradually reduced over a 3-4 week period, before a predetermined cut-off date after which no cigarettes are smoked. The use of nicotine replacement therapy (patches, gum, nasal sprays, and inhalators) can assist greatly in the phased smoking of cigarettes and should be recommended to all smokers. A common programme that health care professionals can recommend:

- Commit to stop: Define and decide specific motivation and desire to stop.
- Discuss medications and strategies to deal with wanting to smoke – maximize success.
- The number of cigarettes/nicotine content should be reduced over a 3–4 week period
- Choose a stop date – complete abstention from that date on.
- Get rid of all tobacco and clean all clothes and car in anticipation of stop date.
- Don't go to places where you would be prone to smoke.
- Ensure and enlist support of co-workers, friends and family to encourage efforts.
- If a parent, realize the example you'll set for your children.
- Don't worry about dieting until safely stopped.

sphygmomanometer long before hospitals adopted it, and accumulated data on hypertension. In 1909, a survey revealed that 22 of the 32 insurance companies were routinely collecting measurement of systolic blood pressure among applicants. These companies, and the doctors they employed, began to conduct the first large-scale surveys of blood pressure, and within just a few years had identified the widespread nature of this asymptomatic problem as well as the existence of isolated systolic hypertension.

It was not until after the Second World War, by which time hospital registries began to show cardiovascular disease as a major cause of mortality, that the rest of the medical community began to accept the importance of hypertension and to conduct epidemiological studies.

The National Heart Institute set up the first long-term epidemiological study of heart 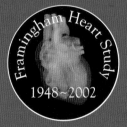 disease in 1948 in the town of Framingham, Massachusetts. More than 5000 men and women aged 30–62 years with no evidence of cardiovascular disease were initially recruited to the survey and followed up by examination every 2 years for 20 years. This prospective epidemiological approach allowed the authors of the Framingham Heart Study to show

Monitoring patients

Depending on blood pressure levels and overall risk for cardiovascular disease, the blood pressure response to non-pharmacological measures should be observed for a variable period. Drug therapy should be introduced more rapidly in patients at high or very high overall risk.
(Fig. 5 Page 37)

Follow-up The frequency of follow-up for treated patients after adequate blood pressure control is attained depends upon factors such as the severity of the hypertension, variability of blood pressure, complexity of the treatment regimen, patient compliance. and the need for non-pharmacological advice. Review every 3 months is sufficient when treatment and blood pressure are stable, and the interval should not generally exceed 6 months. Those who have been hypertensive in the past, or who have untreated mild hypertension and a low estimated 10-year CHD/CVD risk, should have their blood pressure measured and their 10-year CHD/CVD risk estimated annually. The routine for follow-up visits should be simple; measure blood pressure and weight; enquire about general health, side effects and treatment problems; reinforce advice on non-pharmacological measures; and test urine for proteinuria annually. In general practice and hospital clinics trained nurses have an important role in the accurate

conclusively that hypertension is a risk factor for the development of coronary heart disease, stroke and kidney disease.

Framingham paved the way for the era of the controlled clinical trial, which has revolutionized the treatment of hypertension and contributed directly to the decline in death rates from this silent killer.

The era of the controlled clinical trial

In the past 50 years, it is likely that more controlled trials have been conducted in hypertension than in any other disease area, making this the most evidence-based area of medicine. This is clearly a remarkable achievement given that before the introduction of diuretics in the 1950s, there was no effective medical treatment available for hypertension.

In the 1960s, the Veterans' Administration Cooperative Study Group on Antihypertensive Agents established the first randomized, double-blind controlled trials to test the efficacy of antihypertensive drugs in reducing cardiovascular events. These trials showed a significant reduction in stroke and heart failure in patients with severely elevated (115–129 mmHg) or mild to moderately elevated (90–114 mmHg) diastolic blood pressure. It also showed that treatment prevented progression to severe hypertension.

measurement of blood pressure, and can advise and educate patients on aspects such as non-pharmacological measures and possible side effects from drugs. A large proportion of hypertensive patients disappear from regular follow-up for a variety of reasons. This may be reduced by thorough education of the patient about hypertension and its treatment, and provision of written information. A formal system of recall for those who miss routine appointments, using the practice computer, is desirable.

The floodgates had opened and further trials followed, such as the Hypertension Detection and Follow-up Program, confirming the mortality benefits of lowering blood pressure.

In 1990, pooled analyses of nine prospective studies involving 418,343 adults showed that blood pressure levels are positively and continuously related to the risk of having a stroke or a heart attack or of developing heart failure. Furthermore, reducing blood pressure by 10–12 mmHg systolic and 5–6 mmHg diastolic was associated with a 38% reduction in relative risk of stroke and a 16% reduction in relative risk of coronary heart disease.

... *antihypertensive treatment benefits the elderly*

Several trials have now shown the benefits of lowering blood pressure in elderly patients with hypertension, who are particularly prone to isolated systolic hypertension.

Trials such as Systolic Hypertension in the Elderly Programme (SHEP) and Syst-Eur (Systolic Hypertension in Europe) have shown that the elderly benefit particularly in terms of stroke reduction, and that the reduction in blood pressure may also protect patients against vascular dementia.

To date, no trials in the elderly have shown any

Antihypertensive drugs

At present, the available treatment options for hypertension include:

- Diuretics
- Beta-blockers
- Calcium antagonists
- ACE inhibitors
- Angiotensin II antagonists
- Alpha$_1$-blockers

Diuretics Thiazide diuretics are widely available and affordable, and have been shown in controlled trials to improve the prognosis of patients with hypertension, by reducing risk of stroke and CHD. They are reasonably well tolerated, particularly when used at low doses and form part of several combination regimens and fixed-dose combinations. The dose-response curve is relatively flat, so the lowest effective dose should be used. Thiazides are highly effective in older patients with systolic hypertension, as illustrated by the results of the SHEP study.

Although thiazides dominate the anti-hypertensive repertoire, loop diuretics may be preferable in patients with markedly impaired renal function or when fluid retention predominates. Potassium-sparing agents may be considered if there is risk of hypokalaemia.

For cases with resistant hypertension spironolactone is occasionally very effective.

Beta blockers The benefits of these agents in terms of cardiovascular morbidity and mortality

evidence of a reduction in benefits as age increases. The Hypertension in the Very Elderly Trial (HYVET) is currently recruiting patients over 80 years of age to confirm this.

... antihypertensive treatment benefits diabetics

The multicentre UK Prospective Diabetes Study (UKPDS) randomized patients with diabetes to different antihypertensive treatment strategies and showed that tight control of blood pressure (144/82 mmHg) provided significant risk reductions in all diabetes-related endpoints when compared with less tight control of blood pressure (154/87 mmHg).

This was confirmed by the diabetic subgroups of the Hypertension Optimal Treatment (HOT) and the Syst-Eur (Systolic Hypertension in Europe) studies.

... identifying the optimal treatment target

Importantly, large clinical outcome trials have been conducted to provide valuable information on the optimal blood pressure targets that hypertensive therapy should seek to achieve.

The Hypertension Optimal Treatment (HOT)

have been shown in controlled clinical trials albeit to a lesser extent than diuretics. Beta blockers the drug of choice for patients with CHD and are among the most affordable anti-hypertensives. Like diuretics, they may be used in a variety of combination regimens. Heart failure is now an indication for these drugs. However, a decision to initiate therapy in a patient with heart failure should be taken only with caution and may merit consultation with a heart failure specialist.

Beta blockers should not be prescribed for patients with peripheral vascular disease or obstructive airways disease/asthma. Recent evidence suggests the incidence of diabetes may be increased in patients using beta blockers. Beta blockers are less effective in black and older patients.

ACE inhibitors

ACE inhibitors are particularly appropriate for patients with any form of heart failure or left ventricular dysfunction and may be preferred for patients with renal disease, especially when this coincides with diabetes mellitus. These drugs are generally well tolerated; dry cough is the most familiar side effect. Angioedema is a relatively rare but more serious adverse effect that requires immediate action to safeguard the airways. This reaction appears to occur more often in black patients than other races. These agents are more effective in combination with salt restriction and less effective among the elderly.

study enrolled almost 19,000 patients with hypertension from 26 countries and showed that blood pressure levels of 138.5 mmHg systolic and 82.6 mmHg diastolic produced the lowest rate of cardiovascular events. It also confirmed that further lowering of blood pressure was not associated with an increased risk of cardiovascular events.

... newer drugs are as effective as older agents

For many years after the introduction of calcium-channel blockers, ACE inhibitors, alpha-blockers and angiotensin II antagonists, the only real evidence of long-term clinical benefit in terms of reduced mortality and morbidity was available for thiazide diuretics and beta-blockers.

But in recent years, a large number of double-blind outcome studies have been conducted to compare the major classes of antihypertensive drugs. Overall, these have shown no consistent differences in antihypertensive efficacy, side effects or quality of life. A recent meta-analysis by the Blood Pressure Lowering Treatment Triallists' Collaboration looked at the evidence from 17 trials involving 75,924 patients. It confirmed that there is little difference between ACE inhibitors, calcium antagonists and other blood-pressure-lowering drugs on mortality and major cardiovascular morbidity.

Angiotensin II antagonists

These relatively new agents are being extensively scrutinized in controlled trials for their effects on prognosis. Until such studies are completed their principal use is likely to be as alternative therapies for patients who experience dry cough or other adverse effects with ACE inhibitors. However, AIIAs are currently probably the drugs of choice for patients with Type 2 diabetes and proteinuria.

Calcium antagonists

Can be subdivided into 2 major groups – the dihydropyridinies (DHP) (e.g. amlodipine) and the rate limiting group (verapamil and diltiazem). There is good evidence from the Syst-Eur trial that DHPs reduce cardiovascular risk in isolated systolic hypertension – especially the risk of stroke. There has been controversy over the possible adverse effects of calcium antagonists in patients with cardiac ischaemia, but these reservations appear to apply only to short-acting dihydropyridines such as nifedipine which have no place in current therapeutics. So only long-acting calcium antagonists (or sustained action formulations) should be used for hypertension. Calcium antagonists in contrast to beta blockers and ACE inhibitors, are effective, and may be preferred, in black and older patients.

DHP calcium antagonists are generally well tolerated, but may cause ankle oedema, flushes and tachycardia whereas verapamil may cause constipation.

Clinical trials are continuing with several of the agents that are currently available in order to answer the many clinical questions that remain. The Antihypertensive and Lipid-Lowering treatment to prevent Heart Attack Trial (ALLHAT) is the largest study yet conducted on hypertension. The National Heart, Lung, and Blood Institute has enrolled some 40,000 hypertensive subjects over the age of 55 years with at least one additional cardiovascular risk factor. Study drugs include a diuretic (chlorthalidone), a calcium-channel blocker (amlodipine), an ACE inhibitor (lisinopril) and an alpha-blocker (doxasozin). In addition, participants with mild to moderate hypercholesterolaemia have been randomized into an open-label trial designed to determine whether lowering serum cholesterol levels with pravastatin reduces all cause mortality compared with placebo. It is expected that ALLHAT will be completed in 2002.

A further trial is attempting to evaluate the best combination of treatment for patients who require two or more drugs to lower their blood pressure and is also looking at whether the addition of the lipid-lowering agent atorvastatin will give better protection against heart attacks and stroke. The Anglo-Scandinavian Cardiac Outcomes Trial (ASCOT) is comparing combinations of newer antihypertensives (the calcium-channel blocker amlodipine with or without the ACE inhibitor perindopril) to older antihypertensives (the

Alpha blockers

These agents are not generally favoured as first-line therapies because of lack of supportive trial evidence. Their side effects include notably, postural hypotension particularly in the elderly. Recently data from the ALLHAT trial suggested they may increase heart failure if prescribed without diuretics. Their lack of adverse effects on metabolic factors such as lipid and blood glucose may make α blockers a valid treatment option in patients with concomitant disorders such as hyper-lipidaemia, and they are probably the drug of choice for men with concomitant prostatism. These drugs are most commonly used as add-in therapy. Long acting α blockers (e.g doxazosin) are advocated as suitable for men with prostatic hypertrophy.

Centrally-acting agents

Centrally-acting agents are not widely used because their undoubted efficacy as antihypertensives is overshadowed by their unfavourable tolerability profile. Alpha-methyldopa remains the first choice agent in the management of hypertension during pregnancy.

Moxonidine is a recent addition to this group. It has a similar mechanism of action to clonidine but activates imidazoline receptors instead of adrenoceptors and is claimed to have improved tolerability with no reduction in efficacy. They remain unevaluated in any large clinical studies or trials however.

beta-blocker atenolol with or without the diuretic bendroflumethiazide) in reducing the rate of fatal and non-fatal coronary heart disease in 18,000 patients.

International agreement on hypertension and its treatment

As a result of the enormous scientific investment in clinical trials, there is widespread consensus on the definition of hypertension, how it should be measured, the goal of treatment, and the target blood pressure that treatment should achieve.

Guidelines such as those of the World Health Organization (WHO) and the British Hypertension Society define hypertension as a consistent systolic blood pressure above 140 mmHg and diastolic blood pressure above 90 mmHg in people who are not taking antihypertensive medication.

The primary goal of treatment is to achieve the maximum reduction in the total risk of cardiovascular morbidity and mortality by restoring blood pressure to normal or optimal levels.

But increasingly, hypertension experts agree that blood pressure lowering is not the sole aim of treatment. Increasingly, hypertension experts expect treatments to achieve additional

Initiating drug therapy

- Identify factors that favour or oppose the use of particular agents in an individual patient.
- Start with the lowest available dose
- Switch to another *class* of drug, if the response to initial therapy is poor or if treatment is not well tolerated
- If the initial treatment is well tolerated and gives a good but not sufficient response,
  - increase the dose of monotherapy gradually or
  - consider combination therapy
- Try to use drugs that give 24-hour effect from a single daily dose. This gives smooth blood pressure control and encourages good compliance
- The majority of patients will need at least 2 agents

Use of small doses of two or more drugs with complimentary actions may be preferable to large doses of single agents because of better tolerability or reduced potential for untoward metabolic effects (Table 7). Possible drug combinations are listed in Table 8. The new generation of fixed-dose combination preparations that deliver two drugs in a single tablet may help compliance by reducing the number and cost of tablets patients need to take.

Other factors to consider include the possibility of interactions with existing medications, and affordability.

benefits: reducing damage to end organs such as the eyes, kidneys and heart, and preserving organ function. In addition, treatments should reduce coronary risk factors well as improve patients' quality of life.

The British Hypertension Society recommends that antihypertensive treatment be initiated in people with a sustained systolic blood pressure of >160 mmHg or sustained diastolic blood pressure of >100 mmHg. For people with sustained systolic pressure of 140–150 mmHg or sustained diastolic pressure of 90–99 mmHg, treatment decisions should be guided by the presence or absence of target organ damage, cardiovascular disease, diabetes or 10-year coronary heart disease risk >15%.

Treatment should aim for a blood pressure target of <140/85 mmHg. In patients with type 2 diabetes, a lower target of <140/80 mmHg is recommended.

... the story is not over yet

The history of hypertension is a long and distinguished one. Currently available antihypertensive agents have reduced mortality and morbidity from cardiovascular disease, yet the story is far from complete – scientific research continues both in the laboratory and in the clinic.

Indications and contraindications for the major classes of antihypertensive drugs are summarized in Table 8.

Table 7. Metabolic aspects of antihypertensive drugs.

	Beta blockers	Diuretics	Alpha blockers	ACE inhibitors	Calcium antagonists
Fasting insulin	↑	↑	↓	0	0
Fasting blood glucose	↑	(↑)	↓	0	0
Insulin sensitivity	↓	↓	↑	0	0
Total cholesterol	0 (↑)	↑	↓	0	0
HDL	↓	0	↑	0	0
LDL	↑	↑	↓	0	0
TG	↑	↑	↓	0	0

↑ = increase ↓ = decrease 0 = no effect or clinical significance

Table 8. Combination therapies – logical and less logical.

Logical combinations

Thiazide diuretic + beta blocker or ACE inhibitor

Beta blocker + dihydropyridine calcium antagonist

Beta blocker + alpha$_1$ blocker

ACE-inhibitor + calcium antagonist

Less logical combinations

Calcium antagonist + diuretic

Beta blocker + ACE-inhibitor

Combinations to avoid

Beta blocker + non dihydropyridine calcium antagonist
(verapamil or diltiazem)

In many patients, the cause of hypertension remains uncertain. Furthermore, many treated patients still do not achieve a 'normal' blood pressure. So hypertension remains important.

Advances in molecular genetics offer an avenue for further research into the pathophysiology of hypertension through the study of genetic polymorphisms. In addition, there is the prospect that genetic studies may allow the opportunity not only of predicting an individual's risk of developing hypertension, but also their response to antihypertensive lowering treatment, thus allowing preventive treatment to be tailored to specific mechanisms.

While the six currently available classes of antihypertensive agents have brought many benefits, all have disadvantages. So the search for new therapeutic targets continues. New classes of antihypertensives are likely to be available to clinicians over the coming years, notably the neutral endopeptidase inhibitors, which are already being studied in clinical trials.

And, of course, clinical trials such as ALLHAT and ASCOT are continuing in order to provide information regarding the comparative efficacy of different antihypertensive treatment regimens and the additional benefit patients might derive from other means of cardiovascular risk reduction.

Table 9. Guidelines and considerations for the selection of antihypertensive drugs.

Class of drug	Compelling indications	Possible indications	Compelling contra-indications	Possible contra-indications
AIIAs	ACE inhibitor-induced cough[a] Type 2 diabetic nephropathy	Heart failure Intolerance of other anti-hypertensive drugs	Pregnancy Renovascular disease	Renal impairment[c] PVD[b]
ACE inhibitors	Heart failure Left ventricular dysfunction Type 1 diabetic nephropathy	Chronic renal disease[c] Type 2 diabetic nephropathy	Pregnancy Renovascular disease	Renal impairment[c] PVD[b]
Alpha blockers	Prostatism	Dyslipidaemia Sexual dysfunction	Urinary incontinence	Postural hypotension Heart failure
Beta blockers	Myocardial infarction Angina	Heart failure[d]	Asthma/COPD Heart block	Heart failure[d] Dyslipidaemia PVD
Calcium antagonists (DHP)	Elderly ISH	Elderly angina		
Calcium antagonists (rate-limiting)	Angina	Myocardial infarction	Heart block Heart failure Combination with β-blockers	
Diuretics	Elderly ISH Heart failure		Gout	Dyslipidaemia

[a] If ACE inhibitor indicated. [b] Caution with ACE inhibitors and AII antagonists in PVD because of association with renovascular disease. [c] AIIAs and ACE inhibitors may be beneficial in chronic renal failure, but should only be used with caution. Close supervision and specialist advice is required when there is established and significant renal impairment. [d] β-blockers may worsen heart failure, but in special hands may be used to treat heart failure. **ISH = isolated systolic hypertension. COPD = chronic obstructive pulmonary disease.**

References

Blood Pressure Lowering Treatment Triallists'
Collaboration. Effects of ACE inhibitors, calcium
antagonists, and other blood-pressure-lowering drugs:
results of prospectively designed overviews of randomised
trials. *Lancet* 2000; 355: 1955–64.

Bulpitt CJ, Fletcher AE, Amery A et al. The Hypertension in
the Very Elderly Trial (HYVET). Rationale, methodology
and comparison with previous trials. *Drugs Aging* 1994; 5:
171–83.

Collins R, Peto R, MacMahon S et al. Blood pressure,
stroke and coronary heart disease, part 2, short-term
reductions in blood pressure: overview of randomised
drug trials in their epidemiological context. *Lancet* 1990;
325: 827–38.

Hansson L, Zanchetti A, Carruthers SG et al. Effects of
intensive blood pressure lowering and low-dose aspirin in
patients with hypertension: principal results of the HOT
randomised trial. *Lancet* 1998; 351: 1755–62.

Hypertension Detection and Follow-up Program
Cooperative. Five-year findings of the hypertension
detection and follow-up program. 1. Reduction in mortality
of persons with high blood pressure, including mild
hypertension. Hypertension Detection and Follow-up
Program Cooperative Group. *JAMA* 1979; 242: 2562–71.

Kannel WB, Larson M. Long-term epidemiologic prediction
of coronary disease. The Framingham experience.
Cardiology 1993; 82: 137–52.

MacMahon S, Peto R, Cutler J et al. Blood pressure, stroke
and coronary heart disease. Part 1: prolonged differences
in blood pressure: prospective observational studies
corrected for the regression dilution bias. *Lancet* 1990;
335: 765–74.

History checklist

Family history

- [ ] Hypertension
- [ ] Lipid disorder
- [ ] Diabetes
- [ ] Heart attacks
- [ ] Stroke
- [ ] Sudden death

Medical history

- [ ] Angina
- [ ] Stroke
- [ ] Heart failure
- [ ] Previous MI
- [ ] Lipid disorder
- [ ] Claudication

Concomitant disease (affects drug choice)

- [ ] Gout
- [ ] Raynaud's
- [ ] Renal disease
- [ ] Diabetes
- [ ] Asthma

Premenopausal

- [ ] Pregnacy
- [ ] Oral contraceptives

Lifestyle

- [ ] Smoking
- [ ] Alcohol
- [ ] Family situation
- [ ] Exercise
- [ ] Diet/weight
- [ ] Employment
- [ ] Stress
- [ ] Salt

Medication

- [ ] Antidepressants
- [ ] Lithium
- [ ] Nasal decongestants
- [ ] HRT
- [ ] NSAIDs
- [ ] Steriods
- [ ] Cocaine

Symptoms suggesting secondary hypertension

- [ ] Palpitations
- [ ] Panic attacks

Ramsay LE, Williams B, Johnstone DG et al. Guidelines for management of hypertension: report of the third working party of the British Hypertension Society. *J Hum Hypertens* 1999; 13: 569–92.

SHEP Co-operative Research Group. Prevention of stroke by antihypertensive drug treatment in older persons with isolated systolic hypertension. Final results of the Systolic Hypertension in the Elderly Programme. *JAMA* 1991; 265: 3255–64.

Staesson JA, Fagard R, Thijs L et al for the Syst-Eur Trial Investigators. Randomised double-blind comparison of placebo and active treatment for older patients with isolated systolic hypertension. *Lancet* 1997; 350: 757–64.

Tuomilehto J, Rastenyte D, Birkenhager WH et al. Effects of calcium channel blockade in older patients with diabetes and systolic hypertension. Systolic Hypertension in Europe Trial Investigators. *N Engl J Med* 1999; 340: 677–84.

UK Prospective Diabetes Study Group. Tight blood pressure control and risk of macrovascular and microvascular complications in type 2 diabetes: UKPDS 38. *BMJ* 1998; 317: 703–13.

Veterans' Administration Cooperative Study Group on Antihypertensive Agents. Effects of treatment on morbidity in hypertension. Results in patients with diastolic blood pressures averaging 115 through 129 mm Hg. *JAMA* 1967; 202: 1028–34.

Veterans' Administration Cooperative Study Group on Antihypertensive Agents. Effects of treatment on morbidity in hypertension. II. Results in patients with diastolic blood pressure averaging 90 through 114 mm Hg. *JAMA* 1970; 213: 1143–52.

World Health Organization/International Society of Hypertension Guidelines for the management of hypertension. *J Hypertension* 1999; 17: 151–83.

Examination checklist

General features

- [ ] Weight
- [ ] Central obesity
- [ ] Pallor

Eyes

- [ ] Arcus
- [ ] Fundal changes

Neck

- [ ] JVP
- [ ] Thyroid enlarged
- [ ] Carotid bruits

Heart

- [ ] Rate
- [ ] Heave
- [ ] Rhythm
- [ ] Murmurs
- [ ] Displaced
- [ ] Added sounds
- [ ] Ankle oedema
- [ ] Lung fields

Abdomen

- [ ] Liver palpable
- [ ] Aortic pulsation
- [ ] Kidneys
- [ ] Renal bruits
- [ ] Masses

Pulses

- [ ] Femoral delay
- [ ] Femoral bruits
- [ ] Radial delay
- [ ] PVD

Neurology

- [ ] Evidence of stroke

Concomitant disease

- [ ] Asthma
- [ ] Gout
- [ ] Hyperlipidaemia
- [ ] Diabetes

Investigation checklist

- [ ] Urine strip test for blood and protein
- [ ] Blood electrolytes and creatinine
- [ ] Blood glucose
- [ ] Serum total:HDL cholesterol
- [ ] 12 lead electrocardiograph

More detailed investigation should be considered if:

- The history and examination suggests a secondary cause (e.g. coarction)
- The patient is aged less than 40 years
- Hypertension is malignant/severe (DBP >110 mmHg)
- The hypertension is resistant to three or more drugs
- The hypertension is of sudden onset
- There is proteinuria or raised creatinine
- There is hypokalaemia

Secondary causes of hypertension:

- Diabetic nephropathy
- Chronic pyelonephritis
- Obstructive uropathy
- Glomerulonephritis
- Renal artery stenosis
- Polycystic kidneys
- Coarctation of the aorta
- Phaeochromocytoma
- Conn's syndrome
- Cushing's syndrome

Reading

Wood D, Durrington P, Poulter N, McInnes G, Rees A, Wray R on behalf of the British Cardiac Society, British Hyperlipidaemia Association, British Hypertension Society, British Diabetic Association. Joint British recommendations on prevention of coronary heart disease in clinical practice.

Heart 1998; **80** (Suppl. 2).

Raw M, McNeill A, West R. Smoking cessation: evidence-based recommendations for the healthcare system.

Br J Med 1999; **318**: 182–5.

The Guidelines Subcommittee. 1999 World Health Organisation-International Society of Hypertension Guidelines for the Management of Hypertension.

J Hypertens 1999;**17**:151-183.

The Sixth Report of the Joint National Committee on Prevention, Detection, Evaluation, and Treatment of High Blood Pressure.

Arch Intern Med 1997; **157**:2413-2446.

Hansson L *et al* for the HOT Study Group. Effects of intensive blood-pressure lowering and low-dose aspirin in patients with hypertension: principal results of the Hypertension Optimal Treatment (HOT) randomised trial.

Lancet 1998; **351**:1755-1762.

Gress TW *et al*. Hypertension and antihypertensive therapy as risk factors for type 2 diabetes mellitus.

N Engl J Med 2000; **342**:905-912.

Sever PS, Poulter NR. Hypertension drug trials: past present and future.

J Hum Hypertens 2000; **142**:1729-738.

Ramsey LE *et al.* British Hypertension Society National Guidelines for Hypertension Management 1999.
Br Med J 1999; **319**:630-35.

SHEP Cooperative Research group. Prevention of stroke by antihypertensive drug treatment in older persons with isolated systolic hypertension. Final results of the Systolic Hypertension in the Elderly Program (SHEP).
JAMA 1991; **265**:3255-64.

Staessen JA *et al* for the Systolic Hypertension-Europe (Syst-Eur) Trial Investigators. Morbidity and mortality in the placebo-controlled European Trial on Isolated Systolic Hypertension in the Elderly.
Lancet 1997; **350**:757-64.

Literature available from the British Hypertension Society Information Service

E-mail: bhsis@sghms.ac.uk

- **Patient information booklet:**
  - Understanding High Blood Pressure.

- **Patient fact sheets:**
  - Self-help Measures
  - Antihypertensive Drugs
  - Blood Pressure Measurement
  - Reducing Dietary Salt
  - Blood Pressure and Kidney Disease.

- **Diet sheet:**
  - Healthy Eating Diet Sheet.